50 KETO CI
COOKBOOK

Easy and quick delicious chaffle dishes to lose weight fast

Roxana Barbera

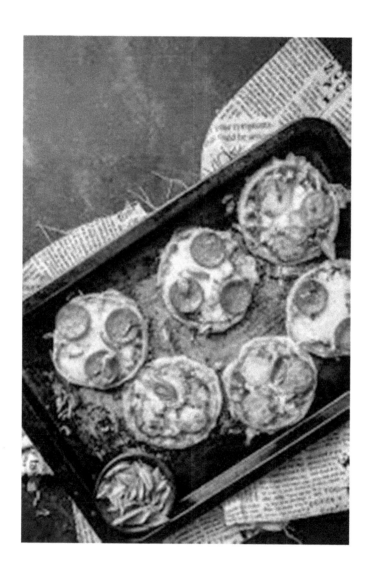

sources. Please consult a licensed professional before attempting any techniques outlined in this book.

By reading this document, the reader agrees that under no circumstances is the author responsible for any losses, direct or indirect, which are incurred as a result of the use of information contained within this document, including, but not limited to, — errors, omissions, or inaccuracies.

TABLE OF CONTENTS

Garlic And Parsley Chaffles

Servings:1

Cooking Time: 5 Minutes

Ingredients:

1 large egg

1/4 cup cheese mozzarella 1 tsp. coconut flour

¼ tsp. baking powder

½ tsp. garlic powder

1 tbsp. minutesced parsley For Serving

1 Poach egg

4 oz. smoked salmon

Directions:

1.   Switch on your Dash waffle maker and let it preheat.

2. Grease waffle maker with cooking spray.

3. Mix egg, mozzarella, coconut flour, baking powder, and garlic powder, parsley to a mixing bowl until combined well.

4. Pour batter in circle chaffle maker.

5. Close the lid.

6. Cook for about 2-3 minutes or until the chaffles are cooked.

7. Serve with smoked salmon and poached egg.

8. Enjoy!

Nutrition Value per Servings: Protein:

140 kcal Fat: 160 kcal Carbohydrates: 14 kcal

Scrambled Eggs On A Spring Onion Chaffle

Servings:4

Cooking Time:7-9 Minutes

Ingredients:

Batter

4 eggs

2 cups grated mozzarella cheese

2 spring onions, finely chopped Salt and pepper to taste

½ teaspoon dried garlic powder 2 tablespoons almond flour

2 tablespoons coconut flour Other

2 tablespoons butter for brushing the waffle maker 6-8 eggs

Salt and pepper

1 teaspoon Italian spice mix 1 tablespoon olive oil

1 tablespoon freshly chopped parsley

Directions:

1.   Preheat the waffle maker.

2.   Crack the eggs into a bowl and add the grated cheese.

3.   Mix until just combined, then add the chopped spring onions and season with salt and pepper and dried garlic powder.

4.   Stir in the almond flour and mix until everything is combined.

5.   Brush the heated waffle maker with butter and add a few tablespoons of the batter.

6.   Close the lid and cook for about 7-8 minutes depending on your waffle maker.

7.   While the chaffles are cooking, prepare the scrambled eggs by whisking the eggs in a bowl until frothy, about 2 minutes. Season with salt and black

pepper to taste and add the Italian spice mix. Whisk to blend in the spices.

8.   Warm the oil in a non-stick pan over medium heat.

9.   Pour the eggs in the pan and cook until eggs are set to your liking.

10.   Serve each chaffle and top with some scrambled eggs. Top with freshly chopped parsley.

Nutrition Value per Servings:

Calories 194, fat 14.7 g, carbs 5 g, Protein 1 g

Strawberry Shortcake Chaffles

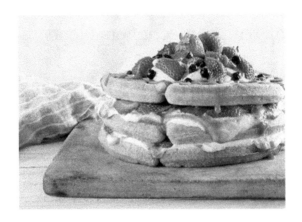

Servings: 1

Prep time: 20 min. Cook time: 25 min.

Ingredients:

FOR THE BATTER:

1 egg

¼ cup mozzarella cheese 1 Tbsp cream cheese

¼ tsp baking powder 2 strawberries, sliced

1 tsp strawberry extract

FOR THE GLAZE:

1 Tbsp cream cheese

¼ tsp strawberry extract

1 Tbsp monk fruit confectioners blend

Directions:

Turn on waffle maker to heat and oil it with cooking spray. Beat egg in a small bowl.

Add remaining batter components. Divide the mixture in half.

Cook one half of the batter in a waffle maker for 4 minutes, or until golden brown. Repeat with remaining batter

Mix all glaze ingredients and spread over each warm chaffle. Mix all whipped cream ingredients and whip until it starts to form peaks. Top each waffle with whipped cream and strawberries.

Nutrition Value per Servings:

Carbs - 5 G Fat - 14 G Protein - 12 G Calories - 218

Glazed Chaffles

Servings: 2

Prep time: 10 min. Cook time: 5 min.

Ingredients:

½ cup mozzarella shredded cheese ⅛ cup cream cheese 2 Tbsp unflavored whey protein isolate

1   Tbsp swerve confectioners sugar substitute ½ tsp baking powder

½ tsp vanilla extract 1 egg

FOR THE GLAZE TOPPING:

2 Tbsp heavy whipping cream

3-4 Tbsp swerve confectioners sugar substitute ½ tsp vanilla extract

Directions:

1. Turn on waffle maker to heat and oil it with cooking spray.

2. In a microwave-safe bowl, mix mozzarella and cream cheese. Heat at 30

3. second intervals until melted and fully combined.

4. Add protein, 2 Tbsp sweetener, baking powder to cheese. Knead with hands until well incorporated. Place dough into a mixing bowl and beat in egg and vanilla until a smooth batter forms.

5. Put ⅓ of the batter into waffle maker, and cook for 3-5 minutes, until golden brown. Repeat until all 3 chaffles are made.

6. Beat glaze ingredients in a bowl and pour over chaffles before serving.

Nutrition Value per Servings:

Carbs - 4 G Fat - 6 G Protein - 4 G Calories – 130

Cream Mini-Chaffles

Servings: 2

Prep time: 5 min. Cook time: 10 min.

Ingredients:

2 tsp coconut flour

4 tsp swerve/monk fruit

¼ tsp baking powder 1 **egg**

1 oz cream cheese

½ tsp vanilla extract

Directions:

1.   Turn on waffle maker to heat and oil it with cooking spray.

2.   Mix swerve/monk fruit, coconut flour, and baking powder in a small mixing bowl. Add cream

cheese, egg, vanilla extract, and whisk until well-combined.

3. Add batter into waffle maker and cook for 3-4 minutes, until golden brown. Serve with your favorite toppings.

Nutrition Value per Servings:

Carbs - 4 G Fat - 6 G Protein - 2 G Calories – 73

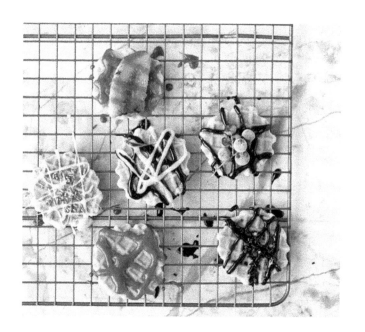

Lemon Curd Chaffles

Servings: 1

prep time: 45 min. Cook time: 5 min.

Ingredients:

3   large eggs

4   oz cream cheese, softened 1 Tbsp low carb sweetener 1 tsp vanilla extract

¾ cup mozzarella cheese, shredded 3 Tbsp coconut flour

1 tsp baking powder

⅓ tsp salt

FOR THE LEMON CURD:

½-1 cup water 5 egg yolks

½ cup lemon juice

½ cup powdered sweetener 2 Tbsp fresh lemon zest

1 tsp vanilla extract Pinch of salt 8 Tbsp cold butter, cubed

Directions:

1. Pour water into a saucepan and heat over medium until it reaches a soft boil. Start with ½ cup and add more if needed.

2. Whisk yolks, lemon juice, lemon zest, powdered sweetener, vanilla, and salt in a medium heat-proof bowl. Leave to set for 5-6 minutes.

3. Place bowl onto saucepan and heat. The bowl shouldn't be touching water. Whisk mixture for 8-10 minutes, or until it begins to thicken.

4. Add butter cubes and whisk for 5-7 minutes, until it thickens. When it lightly coats the back of a spoon, remove from heat. Refrigerate until cool, allowing it to continue thickening.

5. Turn on waffle maker to heat and oil it with cooking spray.

6.   Add baking powder, coconut flour, and salt in a small bowl. Mix well and set aside.

7.   Add eggs, cream cheese, sweetener, and vanilla in a separate bowl. Using a hand beater, beat until frothy.

8.   Add mozzarella to egg mixture and beat again. Add dry ingredients and mix until well-combined.

9.   Add batter to waffle maker and cook for 3-4 minutes. Transfer to a plate and top with lemon curd before serving

Nutrition Value per Servings:

Carbs - 6 G Fat - 24 G Protein - 15 G Calories -302

Egg On A Cheddar Cheese Chaffle

Servings:4

Cooking Time:7-9 Minutes

Ingredients:

Batter 4 eggs

2   cups shredded white cheddar cheese Salt and pepper to taste

2 tablespoons butter for brushing the waffle maker

4 large eggs

2 tablespoons olive oil

Directions:

1.   Preheat the waffle maker.

2.   Crack the eggs into a bowl and whisk them with a fork.

3.   Stir in the grated cheddar cheese and season with salt and pepper.

4.   Brush the heated waffle maker with butter and add a few tablespoons of the batter.

5.   Close the lid and cook for about 7-8 minutes depending on your waffle maker.

6.   While chaffles are cooking, cook the eggs.

7.   Warm the oil in a large non-stick pan that has a lid over medium-low heat for 2-3 minutes

8.   Crack an egg in a small ramekin and gently add it to the pan. Repeat the same way for the other 3 eggs.

9.   Cover and let cook for 2 to 2 ½ minutes for set eggs but with runny yolks.

10.   Remove from heat.

11. To serve, place a chaffle on each plate and top with an egg. Season with salt and black pepper to taste.

Nutrition Value per Servings: Calories 4 fat 34 g, carbs 2 g, sugar 0.6 g, Protein 26 g

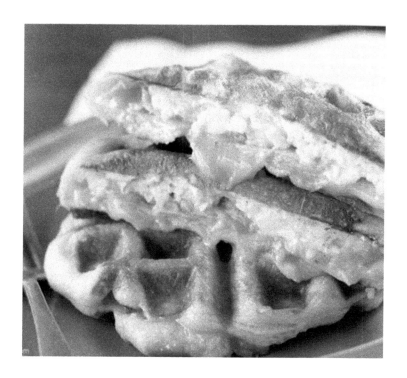

Avocado Chaffle Toast

Servings:3

Cooking Time: 10 Minutes

Ingredients:

4 tbsps. avocado mash 1/2 tsp lemon juice

1/8 tsp salt

1/8 tsp black pepper 2 eggs

1/2 cup shredded cheese For serving

3 eggs

½ avocado thinly sliced 1 tomato, sliced

Directions:

1.   Mash avocado mash with lemon juice, salt, and black pepper in mixing bowl, until well.

2.   In a small bowl beat egg and pour eggs in avocado mixture and mix well.

3.   Switch on Waffle Maker to pre-heat.

4.   Pour 1/8 of shredded cheese in a waffle maker and then pour ½ of egg and avocado mixture and then 1/8 shredded cheese.

5.   Close the lid and cook chaffles for about 3 - 4 minutes.

6.   Repeat with the remaining mixture.

7.   Meanwhile,fry eggs in a pan for about 1-2 minutes.

8.   For serving, arrange fried egg on chaffle toast with avocado slice and tomatoes.

9.   Sprinkle salt and pepper on top and enjoy! Nutrition Value per Servings :

Protein: 66 kcal Fat: 169 kcal Carbohydrates: 15 kcal

Cajun & Feeta Chaffles

Servings:1

Cooking Time: 10 Minutes

Ingredients:

1 egg white

1/4 cup shredded mozzarella cheese 2 tbsps. almond flour

1 tsp Cajun Seasoning FOR SERVING

1 egg

4 oz. feta cheese 1 tomato, sliced

Directions:

1.   Whisk together egg, cheese, and seasoning in a bowl.

2.   Switch on and grease waffle maker with cooking spray.

3.   Pour batter in a preheated waffle maker.

4.   Cook chaffles for about 2-3 minutes until the chaffle is cooked through.

5.   Meanwhile, fry the egg in a non-stick pan for about 1-2 minutes.

6.   For serving set fried egg on chaffles with feta cheese and tomatoes slice. Nutrition Value per Servings:

Protein: 119 kcal Fat 2 kcal Carbohydrates: 31 kcal

Crispy Chaffles With Sausage

Servings:2

Cooking Time: 10 Minutes

Ingredients:

1/2 cup cheddar chease 1/2 tsp. baking powder 1/4 cup egg whites

2 tsp. pumpkin spice 1 egg, whole

2 chicken sausage

2 slice bacon

salt and pepper to taste 1 tsp. avocado oil

Directions:

1.   Mix all ingredients in a bowl.

2.   Allow batter to sit while waffle iron warms.

3.   Spray waffle iron with nonstick spray.

4. Pour batter in the waffle maker and cook according to the directions of the manufacturer.

5. Meanwhile, heat oil in a pan and fry the egg, according to your choice and transfer it toa plate.

6. In the same pan, fry bacon slice and sausage on medium heat for about 2- 3 minutes until cooked.

7. Once chaffles are cooked thoroughly, remove them from the maker.

8. Serve with fried egg, bacon slice, sausages and enjoy! Nutrition Value per Servings:

Calories 208 Fat 13.5g Carbohydrate 0.7g Protein 8.2g Sugars 0.6g

Chili Chaffle

Servings:4

Cooking Time:7-9 Minutes

Ingredients:

Batter 4 eggs

½ cup grated parmesan cheese

1½ cups grated yellow cheddar cheese 1 hot red chili pepper

Salt and pepper to taste

½ teaspoon dried garlic powder 1 teaspoon dried basil

2 tablespoons almond flour Other

2 tablespoons olive oil for brushing the waffle maker

Directions:

1.   Preheat the waffle maker.

2.   Crack the eggs into a bowl and add the grated parmesan and cheddar cheese.

3.   Mix until just combined and add the chopped chili pepper. Season with salt and pepper, dried garlic powder and dried basil. Stir in the almond flour.

4.   Mix until everything is combined.

5.   Brush the heated waffle maker with olive oil and add a few tablespoons of the batter.

6.   Close the lid and cook for about 7-8 minutes depending on your waffle maker.

Nutrition Value per Servings: Calories 36 fat 30.4 g, carbs 3.1 g

Simple Savory Chaffle

Servings:4

Cooking Time: 7-9 Minutes

Ingredients:

Batter 4 eggs

1 cup grated mozzarella cheese

cup grated provolone cheese ½ cup almond flour 2 tablespoons coconut flour

2½ teaspoons baking powder Salt and pepper to taste Other

tablespoons butter to brush the waffle maker

Directions:

1.   Preheat the waffle maker.

2.   Add the grated mozzarella and provolone cheese to a bowl and mix.

3.   Add the almond and coconut flour and baking powder and season with salt and pepper.

4.   Mix with a wire whisk and crack in the eggs.

5.   Stir everything together until batter forms.

6.   Brush the heated waffle maker with butter and add a few tablespoons of the batter.

7.   Close the lid and cook for about 8 minutes depending on your waffle maker.

8.   Serve and enjoy. Nutrition value per Servings:

Calories 352, fat 27.2 g, carbs 8.3 g, Protein 15 g

Pizza Chaffle

Servings:4

Cooking Time:7-9 Minutes

Ingredients:

Batter 4 eggs

1½ cups grated mozzarella cheese

½ cup grated parmesan cheese

2 tablespoons tomato sauce ¼ cup almond flour 1½ teaspoons baking powder

Salt and pepper to taste

teaspoon dried oregano

¼ cup sliced salami Other

tablespoons olive oil for brushing the waffle maker ¼ cup tomato sauce for serving

Directions:

1.   Preheat the waffle maker.

2.   Add the grated mozzarella and grated parmesan to a bowl and mix.

3.   Add the almond flour and baking powder and season with salt and pepper and dried oregano.

4.   Mix with a wooden spoon or wire whisk and crack in the eggs.

5.   Stir everything together until batter forms.

6.   Stir in the chopped salami.

7.   Brush the heated waffle maker with olive oil and add a few tablespoons of the batter.

8.   Close the lid and cook for about 7-minutes depending on your waffle maker.

9.   Serve with extra tomato sauce on top and enjoy. Nutrition value per Servings:

Calories 319, fat 25.2 g, carbs 5.9 g, Protein 19.3 g

Bacon Chaffle

Servings:4

Cooking Time:7-9 Minutes

Ingredients:

Batter 4 eggs

2 cups shredded mozzarella

2 ounces finely chopped bacon Salt and pepper to taste 1 teaspoon dried oregano

Other

2 tablespoons olive oil for brushing the waffle maker

Directions:

1.   Preheat the waffle maker.

2.	Crack the eggs into a bowl and add the grated mozzarella cheese.

3.	Mix until just combined and stir in the chopped bacon.

4.	Season with salt and pepper and dried oregano.

5.	Brush the heated waffle maker with olive oil and add a few tablespoons of the batter.

6.	Close the lid and cook for about 7-8 minutes depending on your waffle maker.

Nutrition value per Servings:

Calories 241, fat 19.8 g, carbs 1.3 g, Protein 14.8 g

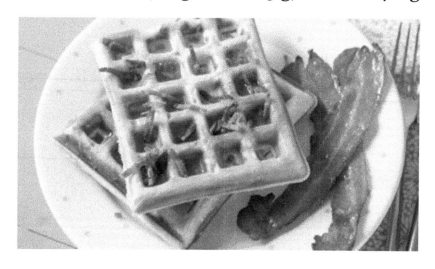

Chaffles Breakfast Bowl

Servings:2

Cooking Time: 5 Minutes

Ingredients:

1 egg

1/2 cup cheddar cheese shredded pinch of Italian seasoning 1 tbsp. pizza sauce

TOPPING:

1/2 avocado sliced 2 eggs boiled

1 tomato, halves

4 oz. fresh spinach leaves

Directions:

1.   Preheat yourwaffle maker and grease with cooking spray.

2.	Crack an egg in a small bowl and beat with Italian seasoning and pizza sauce.

3.	Add shredded cheese to the egg and spices mixture.

4.	Pour 1 tbsp. shredded cheese in a waffle maker and cook for 30 sec.

5.	Pour Chaffles batter inthe waffle maker and close the lid.

6.	Cook chaffles for about 4 minutes until crispy and brown.

7.	Carefully remove chaffles from the maker.

8.	Serve on the bed of spinach with boil **egg,** avocado slice, and tomatoes.

9.	Enjoy!

Nutrition value per Servings:

Protein: 77 kcal Fat: 222 kcal Carbohydrates: 39 kcal

Morning Chaffles With Berries

Servings: 4

Cooking Time: 5 Minutes

Ingredients:

1 cup egg whites

1 cup cheddar cheese, shredded ¼ cup almond flour

¼ cup heavy cream

TOPPING:

4 oz. raspberries

4 oz. strawberries.

1 oz. keto chocolate flakes 1 oz. feta cheese.

Directions:

1.   Preheat your square waffle maker and grease with cooking spray.

2.   Beat egg white in a small bowl with flour.

3.   Add shredded cheese to the egg whites and flour mixture and mix well.

4.   Add cream and cheese tothe egg mixture.

5.   Pour Chaffles batter in a waffle maker and close the lid.

6.   Cook chaffles for about 4 minutes until crispy and brown.

7.   Carefully remove chaffles from the maker.

8.   Serve with berries, cheese, and chocolate on top.

9.   Enjoy!

Nutrition value per Servings:

Protein: 68 kcal Fat: 163 kcal Carbohydrates: 12 kcal

Chocolate Vanilla Chaffles

Servings: 2

Prep time: 5 min. Cook time: 5 min.

Ingredients:

½ cup shredded mozzarella cheese 1 egg

1 Tbsp granulated sweetener 1 tsp vanilla extract

1 Tbsp sugar-free chocolate chips 2 Tbsp almond meal/flour

Directions:

1.   Turn on waffle maker to heat and oil it with cooking spray. Mix all components in a bowl until combined.

2.   Pour half of the batter into waffle maker.

3.   Cook for 2-4 minutes, then remove and repeat with remaining batter. Top with more chips and favorite toppings.

Nutrition Value per Servings:

Carbs - 23 G Fat - 3 G Protein - 4 G Calories – 134

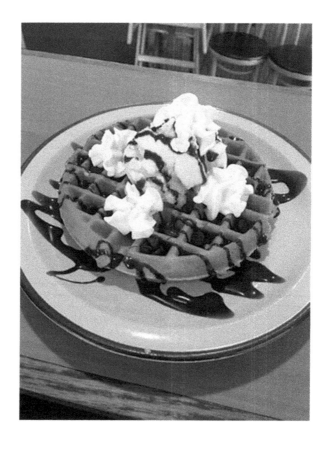

Keto Chaffle Breakfast Sandwich

Prep Time: 3 minutes Cook Time: 6 minutes Servings: 1

Ingredients:

1   egg

1/2 cup Monterey Jack Cheese 1 tablespoon almond flour

2   tablespoons butter

Directions:

1.   In a small bowl, mix the egg, almond flour, and Monterey Jack Cheese.

2.   Pour half of the batter into your mini waffle maker and cook for 3-4 minutes.

3.   Then cook the rest of the batter to make a second chaffle.

4.   In a small pan, melt 2 tablespoons of butter. Add the chaffles and cook on each side for 2 minutes. Pressing down while they are cooking lightly on the top of them, so they crisp up better.

5.   Nutritional Value (per serving):

6.   Calories: 514kcal Carbohydrates: 2g Protein: 21g Fat: 47g

Fudgy Chocolate Chaffles

Servings: 2

Ingredients:

1   egg

2   tbsp mozzarella cheese, shredded

2 tbsp cocoa

2 tbsp Lakanto monk fruit powdered 1 tsp coconut flour

1 tsp heavy whipping cream 1/4 tsp baking powder

1/4 tsp vanilla extract pinch of salt

Directions:

1   Turn on waffle or chaffle maker. I use the Dash Mini Waffle Maker. Grease lightly or use a cooking spray.

2   In a small bowl, combine all ingredients.

3   Cover the dash mini waffle maker with 1/2 of the batter. Close the mini waffle maker and cook for minutes. Remove the chaffle from the waffle maker carefully as it is very hot. Repeat the steps above.

4   Serve with sugar-free strawberry ice cream or sugar-free whipped topping.

Nutritional Value (per serving):

Calories: 109kcal Carbohydrates: 5g Protein: 7g Fat: 7g

Banana Nut Chaffle Recipe

Servings: 2

Ingredients:

1 egg

1 tbs cream cheese, softened and room temp

1 tbs sugar-free cheesecake pudding optional ingredient because it is dirty keto 1/2 cup mozzarella cheese

1 tbs Monkfruit confectioners 1/4 tsp vanilla extract 1/4 tsp banana extract

Optional Toppings: Sugar-free caramel sauce Pecans

Directions:

1   Preheat the mini waffle maker In a small bowl, whip the egg.

2   Add the remaining ingredients to the egg mixture and mix it until it's well incorporated.

3   Add half the batter to the waffle maker and cook it for a minimum of 4 minutes until it's golden brown.

4   Remove the finished chaffle and add the other half of the batter to cook the other chaffle. Top with your optional ingredients and serve warm!

5   Enjoy!

Nutritional Value (per serving):

Total Fat: 7.8g Total Carbohydrate: 2.7g Protein: 8.8g

Chaffle Churros

Servings: 2

Prep time: 10 min. Cook time: 5 min.

Ingredients:

1 egg

1 Tbsp almond flour

½ tsp vanilla extract

1 tsp cinnamon, divided

¼ tsp baking powder

½ cup shredded mozzarella

2 Tbsp swerve brown sugar substitute

1 Tbsp butter, melted

Directions:

1   Turn on waffle maker to heat and oil it with cooking spray.

2   Mix egg, flour, vanilla extract, ½ tsp cinnamon, baking powder, mozzarella, and sugar substitute in a bowl.

3   Place half of the mixture into waffle maker and cook for 3-5 minutes, or until desired doneness. Remove and place the second half of the batter into the maker.

4   Cut chaffles into strips.

5   Place strips in a bowl and cover with melted butter.

6   Mix brown sugar substitute and the remaining cinnamon in a bowl.

7   Pour sugar mixture over the strips and toss to coat them well.

Nutrition Value per Servings:

Carbs - 5 G Fat - 6 G Protein - 5 G Calories – 76

Peanut Butter Chaffle

Servings: 2

Prep time: 5 min. Cook time: 5 min

Ingredients:

1 egg

1 Tbsp heavy cream

1 Tbsp unsweetened cocoa

1 Tbsp lakanto powdered sweetener 1 tsp coconut flour

½ tsp vanilla extract

½ tsp cake batter flavor

¼ tsp baking powder

FOR THE FILLING:

3 Tbsp all-natural peanut butter

2 tsp lakanto powdered sweetener 2 Tbsp heavy cream

Directions:

1   Turn on waffle maker to heat and oil it with cooking spray. Mix all chaffle components in a small bowl.

2   Pour half of the mixture into waffle maker. Cook for 3-5 minutes. Remove and repeat for remaining batter.

3   Allow chaffles to sit for 4-5 minutes so that they crisp up.

4   Mix filling ingredients together and spread it between chaffles. Nutrition Value per Servings:

Carbs - 7 G Fat - 21 G Protein - 9 G Calories – 264

Cinnamon Pecan Chaffles

Servings: 1

Prep time: 20 min. + 12 h. Cook time: 40 min.

Ingredients:

1 Tbsp butter

1   egg

½ tsp vanilla

2   Tbsp almond flour 1 Tbsp coconut flour

⅛ tsp baking powder 1 Tbsp monk fruit

FOR THE CRUMBLE:

½ tsp cinnamon

1 Tbsp melted butter 1 tsp monk fruit

1 Tbsp chopped pecans

Directions:

1   Turn on waffle maker to heat and oil it with cooking spray. Melt butter in a bowl, then mix in the egg and vanilla.

2   Mix in remaining chaffle ingredients.

3   Combine crumble ingredients in a separate bowl.

4   Pour half of the chaffle mix into waffle maker. Top with half of crumble mixture. Cook for 5 minutes, or until done.

5   Repeat with the other half of the batter. Nutrition Value per Servings:

Carbs - 8 G Fat - 35 G Protein - 10 G Calories – 391

Almond Flour Chaffles

Servings: 2

Prep time: 10 min. Cook time: 20 min.

Ingredients:

1 large egg

1 Tbsp blanched almond flour ¼ tsp baking powder

½ cup shredded mozzarella cheese

Directions:

1   Whisk egg, almond flour, and baking powder together. Stir in mozzarella and set batter aside.

2   Turn on waffle maker to heat and oil it with cooking spray.

3   Pour half of the batter onto waffle maker and spread it evenly with a spoon. Cook for 3 minutes, or until it reaches desired doneness.

4   Transfer to a plate and repeat with remaining batter. Let chaffles cool for 2-3 minutes to crisp up.

Nutrition Value per Servings:

Carbs - 2 G Fat - 13 G Protein - 10 G Calories – 131

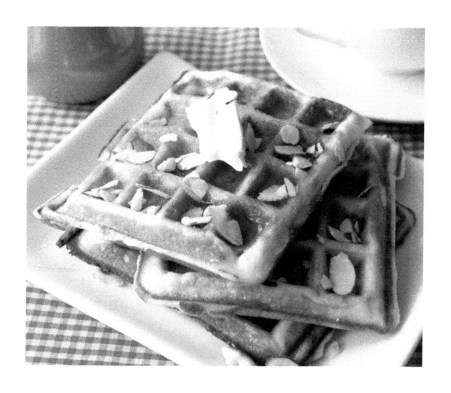

Oreo Keto Chaffles

Servings: 2

Prep time: 5 min. Cook time: 5 min.

Ingredients:

1   egg

1½ Tbsp unsweetened cocoa

2   Tbsp lakanto monk fruit, or choice of sweetener 1 Tbsp heavy cream

1 tsp coconut flour

½ tsp baking powder

½ tsp vanilla

FOR THE CHEESE CREAM:

1   Tbsp lakanto powdered sweetener

2   Tbsp softened cream cheese ¼ tsp vanilla

Directions:

1   Turn on waffle maker to heat and oil it with cooking spray. Combine all chaffle ingredients in a small bowl.

2   Pour one half of the chaffle mixture into waffle maker. Cook for 3-5 minutes.

3   Remove and repeat with the second half if the mixture. Let chaffles sit for 2-3 to crisp up.

4   Combine all cream ingredients and spread on chaffle when they have cooled to room temperature.

Nutrition Value per Servings:

Carbs - 3 G Fat - 4 G Protein - 7 G Calories – 66

Chicken Bites With Chaffles

Servings: 2

Cooking Time: 10 minutes

Ingredients:

1 chicken breastscut into 2 x2 inch chunks 1 egg, whisked

1/4 cup almond flour 2 tbsps. onion powder 2 tbsps. garlic powder 1 tsp. dried oregano

1 tsp. paprika powder 1 tsp. salt

1/2 tsp. black pepper 2 tbsps. avocado oil

Directions:

1.   Add all the dry ingredients together into a large bowl.Mix well.

2.   Place the eggs into a separate bowl.

3.   Dip each chicken piece into the egg and then into the dry ingredients.

4.   Heat oil in 10-inch skillet, add oil.

5.   Once avocado oil is hot, place the coated chicken nuggets onto a skillet and cook for 6-8 minutes until cooked and golden brown.

6.   Serve with chaffles and raspberries.

7.   Enjoy!

Nutrition value per Servings: :

Calories 401 Kcal Fats 219 G Protein 32.35 G Net Carbs 1.46 G

Crunchy Fish And Chaffle Bites

Servings:4

Cooking Time: 15 Minutes

Ingredients:

1 lb. cod fillets, sliced into 4 slice 1 tsp. sea salt

1 tsp. garlic powder 1 egg, whisked

1   cup almond flour 2 tbsp. avocado oil

CHAFFLE Ingredients:

2   eggs

1/2 cup cheddar cheese 2 tbsps. almond flour

½ tsp. Italian seasoning

Directions:

1.   Mix chaffle ingredients in a bowl and make 4 square

2.   Put the chaffles in a preheated chaffle maker.

3.   Mix the salt, pepper, and garlic powder in a mixing bowl. Toss the cod cubes in this mixture and let sit for 10 minutes.

4.   Then dip each cod slice into the egg mixture and then into the almond flour.

5.   Heat oil in skillet and fish cubes for about 2-3 minutes, until cooked and browned

6.   Serve on chaffles and enjoy! Nutrition value perServings:

Protein: 38% 121 Kcal Fat: 59% 189 Kcal Carbohydrates: 3% 11 Kcal

Grill Pork Chaffle Sandwich

Servings:2

Cooking Time: 15 Minutes

Ingredients:

1/2 cup mozzarella, shredded 1 egg

I pinch garlic powder PORK PATTY

1/2 cup pork, minutesced 1 tbsp. green onion, diced 1/2 tsp Italian seasoning Lettuce leaves

Directions:

1.   Preheat the square waffle maker and grease with

2.   Mix egg, cheese and garlic powder in a small mixing bowl.

3.   Pour batter in a preheated waffle maker and close the lid.

4.   Make 2 chaffles from thisbatter.

5.   Cook chaffles for about 2-3 minutes until cooked through.

6.   Meanwhile, mix pork patty ingredients in a bowl and make 1 large patty.

7.   Grill pork patty in a preheated grill for about 3-4 minutes per side until cooked through.

8.   Arrange pork patty between two chaffles with lettuce leaves. Cut sandwich to make a triangular sandwich.

9.   Enjoy!

Nutrition value per Servings:

Protein: 85 Kcal Fat: 86 Kcal Carbohydrates: 7 Kcal

Chaffle & Chicken Lunch Plate

Servings:1

Cooking Time: 15 Minutes

Ingredients:

1 large egg

1/2 cup jack cheese, shredded 1 pinch salt

For Serving 1 chicken leg salt

pepper

1 tsp. garlic, minutesced 1 egg

I tsp avocado oil

Directions:

1.   Heat your square waffle maker and grease with cooking spray.

2. Pour Chaffle batter intothe skillet and cook for about 3 minutes.

3. Meanwhile,heat oil in a pan, over medium heat.

4. Once the oil is hot, add chicken thigh and garlicthen, cook for about 5 minutes. Flip and cook for another 3-4 minutes.

5. Season with salt and pepper and give them a good mix.

6. Transfer cooked thigh to plate.

7. Fry the egg in the same pan for about 1-2 minutes according to your choice.

8. Once chaffles are cooked, serve with fried egg and chicken thigh

9. Enjoy!

Nutrition value per Servings:

Protein: 31% 138 Kcal Fat: 66% 292 Kcal Carbohydrates: 2% Kcal

Keto Blt Chaffle Sandwich

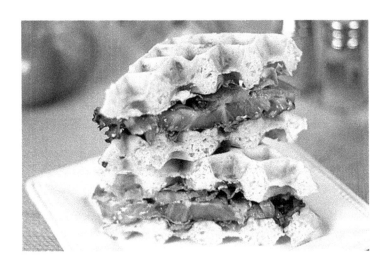

Ingredients:

Chaffle bread ingredients:

1/2 cup mozzarella shredded 1 egg

1 tbs green onion diced 1/2 tsp Italian seasoning Sandwich ingredients:

Bacon pre-cooked Lettuce

Tomato sliced 1 tbs mayo

Directions:

1   Preheat the mini waffle maker In a small bowl, whip the egg.

2   Add the cheese, seasonings, and onion. Mix it until it's well incorporated. Place half the batter in the mini waffle maker and cook it for 4 minutes.

3   If you want a crunchy bread, add a tsp of shredded cheese to the mini waffle iron for 30 seconds before adding the batter. The extra cheese on the outside creates the best crust!

4   After the first chaffle is complete, add the remaining batter to the mini waffle maker and cook it for 4 minutes.

5   Add the mayo, bacon, lettuce, and tomato to your sandwich. Enjoy!

Lime Pie Chaffle Recipe

Servings: 2

Ingredients:

Key Lime Pie Chaffle Recipe ingredients:

1   egg

1/4 cup Almond flour

2   tsp cream cheese room temp

1 tsp powdered sweetener swerve or monk fruit

1/2 tsp lime extract or 1 tsp fresh squeezed lime juice 1/2 tsp baking powder 1/2 tsp lime zest

Pinch of salt to bring out the flavors Cream Cheese Lime Frosting Ingredients:

4 oz cream cheese softened 4 tbs butter

2 tsp powdered sweetener swerve or monk fruit 1 tsp lime extract

1/2 tsp lime zest

Directions:

1   Preheat the mini waffle iron.

2   In a blender, add all the chaffle ingredients and blend on high until the mixture is smooth and creamy.

3   Cook each chaffle about 3 to 4 minutes until it's golden brown. While the chaffles are cooking, make the frosting.

4   In a small bowl, combine all the ingredients for the frosting and mix it until it's smooth. Allow the chaffles to completely cool before frosting them.

Optional:

Top with whipped cream or the cream cheese frosting. Add a small amount

of lime zest for an extra touch!

Nutritional Value (per serving):

Total Fat 5.7g Total Carbohydrate 4.9g Protein 5.5g

Easy Turkey Burger With Halloumi Cheese Chaffle Recipe

Servings 4

Ingredients:

1 lb Ground Turkey raw (no need to precook the turkey) 8 oz Halloumi shredded

1 zucchini medium, shredded 2 tbsp Chives chopped

1/2 tsp Salt1/4 tsp Pepper

Directions:

1   Add all ingredients to a bowl mix thoroughly together. Shape into 8 evenly sized patties.

2   Preheat mini griddle.

3   Cook the patties for 5-7 minutes.

Nutritional Value (per serving):

Calories 222 Total Fat 18g Total Carbohydrate 0.3g
Protein 14.2g

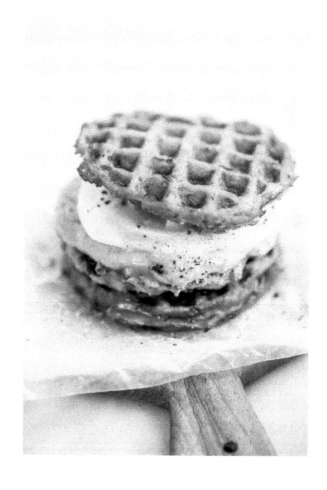

Gingerbread Chaffle

Servings: 2

Prep time: 5 min. Cook time: 5 min.

Ingredients:

½ cup mozzarella cheese grated 1 medium egg

½ tsp baking powder

1 tsp erythritol powdered

½ tsp ground ginger

¼ tsp ground nutmeg

½ tsp ground cinnamon

⅛ tsp ground cloves 2 Tbsp almond flour

1   cup heavy whipped cream

¼ cup keto-friendly maple syrup

Directions:

1   Turn on waffle maker to heat and oil it with cooking spray. Beat egg in a bowl.

2   Add flour, mozzarella, spices, baking powder, and erythritol. Mix well. Spoon one half of the batter into waffle maker and spread out evenly.

3   Close and cook for 5 minutes.

4   Remove cooked chaffle and repeat with remaining batter. Serve with whipped cream and maple syrup.

Nutrition Value per Servings:

Carbs - 5 G Fat - 15 G Protein - 12 G Calories – 103

Chocolate Peanut Butter Chaffle

Servings: 2

Prep time: 5 min. Cook time: 10 min

Ingredients:

½ cup shredded mozzarella cheese 1 Tbsp cocoa powder

2 Tbsp powdered sweetener 2 Tbsp peanut butter

½ tsp vanilla 1 egg

2 Tbsp crushed peanuts 2 Tbsp whipped cream

¼ cup sugar-free chocolate syrup

Directions:

1   Combine mozzarella, egg, vanilla, peanut butter, cocoa powder, and sweetener in a bowl. Add in peanuts and mix well.

2   Turn on waffle maker and oil it with cooking spray.

3   Pour one half of the batter into waffle maker, cook for 4 minutes, and then transfer to a plate. Top with whipped cream, peanuts, and sugar-free chocolate syrup.

Nutrition Value per Servings:

Carbs - 6 G Fat - 17 G Protein - 15 G Calories – 236

Pumpkin Pecan Chaffles

Servings: 2

Prep time: 10 min. Cook time: 10 min.

Ingredients:

1 egg

½ cup mozzarella cheese grated 1 Tbsp pumpkin puree

½ tsp pumpkin spice

1 tsp erythritol low carb sweetener 2 Tbsp almond flour

2 Tbsp pecans, toasted chopped 1 cup heavy whipped cream

¼ cup low carb caramel sauce

Directions:

1   Turn on waffle maker to heat and oil it with cooking spray. In a bowl, beat egg.

2   Mix in mozzarella, pumpkin, flour, pumpkin spice, and erythritol. Stir in pecan pieces.

3   Spoon one half of the batter into waffle maker and spread evenly. Close and cook for 5 minutes.

4   Remove cooked waffles to a plate. Repeat with remaining batter. Serve with pecans, whipped cream, and low carb caramel sauce.

Nutrition Value per Servings:

Carbs - 4 G Fat - 17 G Protein - 11 G Calories – 210

Italian Cream Chaffle Sandwich-Cake

Ingredients:

4 oz cream cheese, softened, at room tempereture 4 eggs

1 Tbsp melted butter 1 tsp vanilla extract

½ tsp cinnamon

1 Tbsp monk fruit sweetener 4 Tbsp coconut flour

1 Tbsp almond flour

1½ teaspoons baking powder

1 Tbsp coconut, shredded and unsweetened 1 Tbsp walnuts, chopped

FOR THE ITALIAN CREAM FROSTING:

2 oz cream cheese, softened, at room temperature 2 Tbsp butter room temp

2 Tbsp monk fruit sweetener ½ tsp vanilla

Directions:

1   Combine cream cheese, eggs, melted butter, vanilla, sweetener, flours, and baking powder in a blender. Add walnuts and coconut to the mixture.

2   Blend to get a creamy mixture.

3   Turn on waffle maker to heat and oil it with cooking spray.

4   Add enough batter to fill waffle maker. Cook for 2-3 minutes, until chaffles are done. Remove and let them cool.

5   Mix all frosting ingredients in another bowl. Stir until smooth and creamy. Frost the chaffles once they have cooled.

6   Top with cream and more nuts

Nutrition Value per Servings:Carbs - 31 G Fat - 2 G Protein - 5 G Calories – 168

Chocolate Cherry Chaffles

Servings: 1

Prep time: 5 min. Cook time: 5 min.

Ingredients:

1 Tbsp almond flour 1 Tbsp cocoa powder

1 Tbsp sugar free sweetener ½ tsp baking powder 1 whole egg

½ cup mozzarella cheese shredded

2 Tbsp heavy whipping cream whipped 2 Tbsp sugar free cherry pie filling

1 Tbsp chocolate chips

Directions:

1 Turn on waffle maker to heat and oil it with cooking spray. Mix all dry components in a bowl.

2   Add egg and mix well.

3   Add cheese and stir again.

4   Spoon batter into waffle maker and close. Cook for 5 minutes, until done. Top with whipping cream, cherries, and chocolate chips.

Nutrition Value per Servings:

Carbs - 6 G Fat - 1 G Protein - 1 G Calories – 130

Banana Nut Chaffle

Servings: 1

Prep time: 15 min.Cook time: 10 min.

Ingredients:

1 egg

1 Tbsp cream cheese, softened and room temp

1 Tbsp sugar-free cheesecake pudding ½ cup mozzarella cheese 1 Tbsp monk fruit confectioners sweetener ¼ tsp vanilla extract

¼ tsp banana extract toppings of choice

Directions:

1 Turn on waffle maker to heat and oil it with cooking spray. Beat egg in a small bowl.

2   Add remaining ingredients and mix until well incorporated.

3   Add one half of the batter to waffle maker and cook for 4 minutes, until golden brown. Remove chaffle and add the other half of the batter.

4   Top with your optional toppings and serve warm!

Nutrition Value per Servings:

Carbs - 2 G Fat - 7 G Protein - 8 G Calories – 119

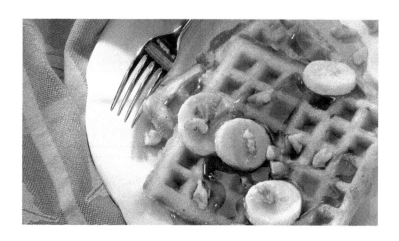

Belgium Chaffles

Servings: 1

Prep time: 5 min. Cook time: 6 min.

Ingredients:

2   eggs

1   cup Reduced-fat Cheddar cheese, shredded

Directions:

1   Turn on waffle maker to heat and oil it with cooking spray.

2   Whisk eggs in a bowl, add cheese. Stir until well-combined.

3   Pour mixture into waffle maker and cook for 6 minutes until done. Let it cool a little to crisp before serving.

Nutrition Value per Servings:

Carbs - 2 G Fat - 33 G Protein - 44 G Calories – 460

Bacon Chaffles

Servings: 2

Prep time: 5 min. Cook time: 5 min.

Ingredients:

2 eggs

½ cup cheddar cheese

½ cup mozzarella cheese

¼ tsp baking powder

½ Tbsp almond flour

1 Tbsp butter, for waffle maker

FOR THE FILLING:

¼ cup bacon, chopped

2 Tbsp green onions, chopped

Directions:

1   Turn on waffle maker to heat and oil it with cooking spray.

2   Add eggs, mozzarella, cheddar, almond flour, and baking powder to a blender and pulse 10 times, so cheese is still chunky.

3   Add bacon and green onions. Pulse 2-3 times to combine.

4   Add one half of the batter to the waffle maker and cook for 3 minutes, until golden brown.

5   Repeat with remaining batter. Add your toppings and serve ot. Nutrition Value per Servings:

Carbs - 3 G Fat - 38 G Protein - 23 G Calories – 446

Chaffle Egg Sandwich

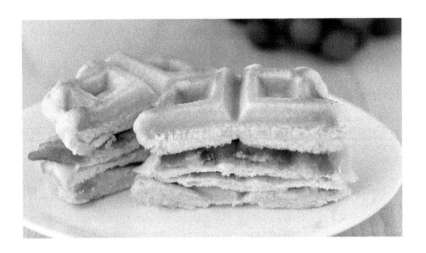

Servings: 2

Cooking Time: 10 Minutes

Ingredients:

2 minutesI keto chaffle

2 slice cheddar cheese 1 egg simple omelet

Directions:

1.   Prepare your oven on 4000 F.

2.   Arrange egg omelet and cheese slice between chaffles.

3.   Bake in the preheated oven for about 4-5 minutes until cheese is melted.

4.   Once the cheese is melted, remove from the oven.

5.   Serve and enjoy! Nutrition value per Servings:

Protein: 144 kcal Fat: 337 kcal Carbohydrates: 14 kcal

Chaffle Minutesi Sandwich

Servings: 2

Cooking Time: 10 Minutes

Ingredients:

1   large egg

1/8 cup almond flour 1/2 tsp. garlic powder 3/4 tsp. baking powder 1/2 cup shredded cheese

SANDWICH FILLING:

2   slices deli ham 2 slices tomatoes

1   slice cheddar cheese

Directions:

1.   Grease your square waffle maker and preheat it on medium heat.

2.   Mix chaffle ingredients in a mixing bowl until well combined.

3.   Pour batter intoa square waffle and make two chaffles.

4.   Once chaffles are cooked, remove from the maker.

5.   For a sandwich,arrange deli ham, tomato slice and cheddar cheese between two chaffles.

6.   Cut sandwich from the center.

7.   Serve and enjoy! Nutrition value per Servings:

Calories 208 Fat 13.5g Carbohydrate 0.7g Protein 8.2g Sugars 0.6g

Chaffle Cheese Sandwich

Servings: 1

Cooking Time: 10 Minutes

Ingredients:

2   square keto chaffle 2 slice cheddar cheese

2 lettuce leaves

Directions:

1.   Prepare your oven on 4000 F.

2.   Arrange lettuce leave and cheese slice between chaffles.

3.   Bake in the preheated oven for about 4-5 minutes until cheese is melted.

4.   Once the cheese is melted, remove from the oven.

5. Serve and enjoy! Nutrition value per Servings:

Calories 208 Fat 13.5g Carbohydrate 0.7g Protein 8.2g Sugars 0.6g

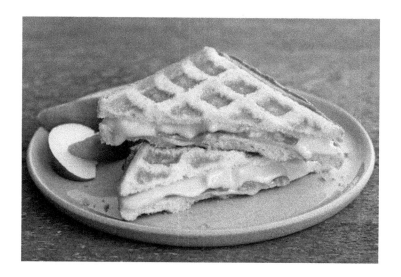

Chicken Zinger Chaffle

Servings:2

Cooking Time: 15 Minutes

Ingredients:

1 chicken breast, cut into 2 pieces 1/2 cup coconut flour 1/4 cup finely grated Parmesan

1 tsp. paprika

1/2 tsp. garlic powder 1/2 tsp. onion powder 1 tsp. salt& pepper

1   egg beaten

Avocado oil for frying Lettuce leaves BBQ sauce

CHAFFLE Ingredients: 4 oz. cheese

2   whole eggs

2 oz. almond flour 1/4 cup almond flour 1 tsp baking powder

Directions:

1.   Mix chaffle ingredients in a bowl.

2.   Pour the chaffle batter in preheated greased square chaffle maker.

3.   Cook chaffles for about 2-minutes until cooked through.

4.   Make square chaffles from this batter.

5.   Meanwhile mix coconut flour, parmesan, paprika, garlic powder, onion powder salt and pepper in a bowl.

6.   Dip chicken first in coconut flour mixture then in beaten egg.

7.   Heat avocado oil in a skillet and cook chicken from both sides. until lightly brown and cooked

8.   Set chicken zinger between two chaffles with lettuce and BBQ sauce.

9.   Enjoy!

Nutrition value per Servings:

Calories 208 Fat 13.5g Carbohydrate 0.7g Protein 8.2g Sugars 0.6g

Double Chicken Chaffles

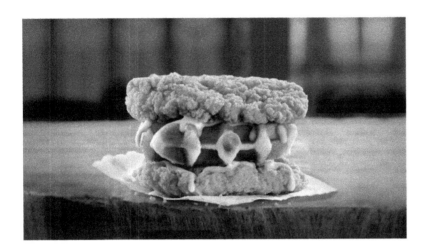

Servings:2

Cooking Time: 5 Minutes

Ingredients:

1/2 cup boil shredded chicken 1/4 cup cheddar cheese

1/8 cup parmesan cheese 1 egg

1 tsp. Italian seasoning

1/8 tsp. garlic powder 1 tsp. cream cheese

Directions:

1.   Preheat the Belgian waffle maker.

2.   Mix in chaffle ingredients in a bowl and mix.

3.   Sprinkle 1 tbsp. of cheese in a waffle maker and pour in chaffle batter.

4.   Pour 1 tbsp. of cheese over batter and close the lid.

5.   Cook chaffles for about 4 to minutes.

6.   Serve with a chicken zinger and enjoy the double chicken flavor. Nutrition value per Servings:

Calories 208 Fat 13.5g Carbohydrate 0.7g Protein 8.2g Sugars 0.6g

Chaffles With Topping

Servings: 3

Cooking Time: 10 Minutes

Ingredients:

1 large egg

1 tbsp. almond flour

1 tbsp. full-fat Greek yogurt 1/8 tsp baking powder

1/4 cup shredded Swiss cheese TOPPING

4oz. grillprawns

4 oz. steamed cauliflower mash 1/2 zucchini sliced
3 lettuce leaves

1 tomato, sliced

1 tbsp. flax seeds

Directions:

1.   Make 3 chaffles with the given chaffles ingredients.

2.   For serving, arrange lettuce leaves on each chaffle.

3.   Top with zucchini slice, grill prawns, cauliflower mash and a tomato slice.

4.   Drizzle flax seeds on top.

5.   Serve and enjoy! Nutrition value per Servings:

Calories 208 Fat 13.5g Carbohydrate 0.7g Protein 8.2g Sugars 0.6g

Chaffle With Cheese & Bacon

Servings:2

Cooking Time: 15 Minutes

ingredients:

1 egg

1/2 cup cheddar cheese, shredded 1 tbsp. parmesan cheese

3/4 tsp coconut flour 1/4 tsp baking powder

1/8 tsp Italian Seasoning pinch of salt

1/4 tsp garlic powder

FOR TOPPING:

1 bacon sliced, cooked and chopped 1/2 cup mozzarella cheese, shredded

1/4 tsp parsley, chopped

Directions:

1.   Preheat oven to 400 degrees.

2.   Switch on your minutesi waffle maker and grease with cooking spray.

3.   Mix chaffle ingredients in a mixing bowl until combined.

4.   Spoon half of the batter in the center of the waffle maker and close the lid. Cook chaffles for about 3-minutes until cooked.

5.   Carefully remove chaffles from the maker.

6.   Arrange chaffles in a greased baking tray.

7.   Top with mozzarella cheese, chopped bacon and parsley.

8.   And bake in the oven for 4 -5 minutes.

9.   Once the cheese is melted, remove from the oven.

10.   Serve and enjoy! Nutrition value per Servings:

Calories 208 Fat 13.5g Carbohydrate 0.7g Protein 8.2g Sugars 0.6g

Grill Beefsteak And Chaffle

Servings: 1

Cooking Time: 10 Minutes

Ingredients:

1 beefsteak rib eye 1 tsp salt

1 tsp pepper

1 tbsp. lime juice 1 tsp garlic

Directions:

1.   Prepare your grill for direct heat.

2.   Mix all spices and rub over beefsteak evenly.

3.   Place the beef on the grill rack over medium heat.

4.   Cover and cook steak for about6 to 8 minutes. Flip and cook for another 5 minutes until cooked through.

5.   Serve with keto simple chaffle and enjoy! Nutrition value per Servings:

Calories 208 Fat 13.5g Carbohydrate 0.7g Protein 8.2g Sugars 0.6g

Cauliflower Chaffles And Tomatoes

Servings:2

Cooking Time: 15 Minutes

Ingredients:

1/2 cup cauliflower 1/4 tsp. garlic powder 1/4 tsp. black pepper 1/4 tsp. Salt

1/2 cup shredded cheddar cheese 1 egg

FOR TOPPING:

1 lettuce leave

1 tomato sliced

4 oz. cauliflower steamed, mashed 1 tsp sesame seeds

Directions:

1.   Add all chaffle ingredients into a blender and mix well.

2.   Sprinkle 1/8 shredded cheese on the waffle maker and pour cauliflower mixture in a preheated waffle maker and sprinkle the rest of the cheese over

it.

3.   Cook chaffles for about 4-5 minutes until cooked

4.   For serving, lay lettuce leaves over chaffle top with steamed cauliflower and tomato.

5.   Drizzle sesame seeds on top.

6.   Enjoy!

Nutrition value per Servings:

Calories 208 Fat 13.5g Carbohydrate 0.7g Protein 8.2g Sugars 0.6g

Layered Cheese Chaffles

Servings: 1

Cooking Time: 5 Minutes

Ingredients:

1   organic egg, beaten

1/3 cup Cheddar cheese, shredded

½ teaspoon ground flaxseed

¼ teaspoon organic baking powder

2   tablespoons Parmesan cheese, shredded

Directions:

1.   Preheat a mini waffle iron and then grease it.

2.   In a bowl, place all the ingredients except Parmesan and beat until well combined.

3.   Place half the Parmesan cheese in the bottom of preheated waffle iron.

4.   Place half of the egg mixture over cheese and top with the remaining Parmesan cheese.

5.   Cook for about 3-minutes or until golden brown.

6.   Serve warm.

Nutrition value per Servings:

Calories 208 Fat 13.5g Carbohydrate 0.7g Protein 8.2g Sugars 0.6g

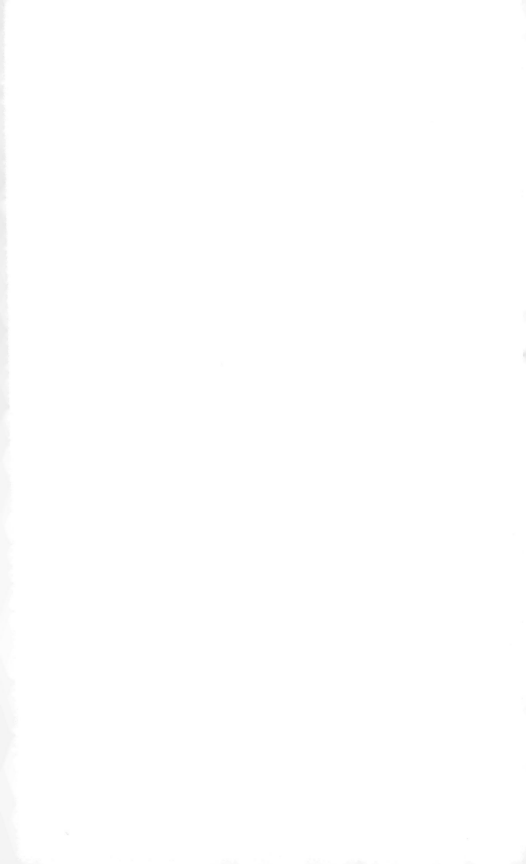

Lightning Source UK Ltd.
Milton Keynes UK
UKHW020656110321
380169UK00012B/890